The Love-Hate Relationship Between Fruit and Diabetics

Introduction

Overview of Diabetes and Diet

Diabetes is a chronic condition that affects millions of people worldwide.

It's characterized by the body's inability to regulate blood sugar levels effectively, leading to a range of health complications if not managed properly.

There are two main types of diabetes: Type 1 and Type 2.

Type 1 diabetes is an autoimmune condition where the body's immune system attacks insulin-producing cells in the pancreas, leading to little or no insulin production.

On the other hand, Type 2 diabetes, which is far more common, occurs when the body becomes resistant to insulin or doesn't produce enough of it.

The management of diabetes largely revolves around controlling blood sugar levels through a combination of medication, exercise, and, most importantly, diet.

The foods diabetics consume have a direct impact on their blood glucose levels, making dietary choices crucial in preventing spikes and maintaining overall health. This brings us to the focal point of our discussion – fruit.

Fruit, often hailed as nature's candy, is packed with vitamins, minerals, antioxidants, and fiber, making it a staple in many healthy diets.

However, for diabetics, fruit represents a complex challenge. While fruits offer numerous health benefits, they also contain natural sugars that can cause blood sugar levels to rise.

This creates a love-hate relationship between fruit and diabetics, where the nutritional benefits must be carefully weighed against the potential risks.

In this extensive discussion, we will explore the intricate dynamics between fruit and diabetes. We'll delve into the reasons why fruit is both cherished and feared by those managing diabetes, examine the nutritional benefits, identify the challenges, and offer practical advice for navigating this love-hate relationship.

Whether you're a diabetic looking to better understand how fruit fits into your diet or someone supporting a loved one with diabetes, this conversation will provide valuable insights and actionable tips.

Diabetes and Diet: A Balancing Act

Living with diabetes means constantly balancing the foods you love with the need to maintain healthy blood sugar levels.

For many diabetics, fruit is a source of both delight and anxiety. On one hand, the vibrant colors, sweet flavors, and health benefits make fruit an attractive choice.

On the other, the natural sugars in fruit can be a source of concern, especially when trying to avoid blood sugar spikes.

Understanding how to include fruit in a diabetic diet requires knowledge of the different types of fruits, their sugar content, and how they interact with the body.

It also involves learning strategies to enjoy fruit in a way that supports rather than undermines diabetes management.

This balance is key to not only managing diabetes effectively but also enjoying a varied and satisfying diet.

In the following chapters, we will explore the many facets of this love-hate relationship, starting with the positive aspects of fruit consumption. From the vitamins and minerals that support overall health to the fiber that helps regulate blood sugar, we'll take a closer look at why fruit deserves a place in the diabetic diet, despite its challenges.

Chapter 1: The Love – Nutritional Benefits of Fruit for Diabetics

Nutrient Density of Fruits

When it comes to managing diabetes, understanding the nutrient composition of the foods you consume is crucial.

Fruits, in particular, are often celebrated for their nutrient density, which means they provide a high amount of essential nutrients relative to their calorie content.

For diabetics, this is a significant factor because it allows for the intake of vital vitamins, minerals, and other compounds without consuming excessive calories or harmful substances.

<u>Vitamins and Minerals</u>

  Fruits are a powerhouse of vitamins and minerals, many of which play a direct role in managing and mitigating the effects of diabetes. For instance:
- Vitamin C:
  Found in abundance in fruits like oranges, strawberries, and kiwi, Vitamin C is not only an antioxidant but also helps improve the body's sensitivity to insulin. Improved insulin sensitivity can help in better glucose management, making it easier for the body to regulate blood sugar levels.

- Potassium:

Bananas, oranges, and melons are rich sources of potassium.

This mineral is essential for maintaining healthy blood pressure levels, which is particularly important for diabetics who are at a higher risk of developing cardiovascular complications.

- Magnesium:

Fruits like bananas, avocados, and figs are rich in magnesium, a mineral that plays a role in over 300 enzymatic reactions in the body, including those involved in glucose regulation and insulin production.

- Fiber:

 While technically not a vitamin
or mineral, fiber is a critical
component found in fruits like
apples, pears, and berries.

 It slows down the absorption of
sugar into the bloodstream,
which helps prevent spikes in
blood sugar levels after eating.

Antioxidants

Antioxidants are compounds that protect the body from oxidative stress, which occurs when there is an imbalance between free radicals and antioxidants in the body.

Oxidative stress is linked to a number of chronic conditions, including diabetes.

Fruits are one of the richest sources of antioxidants, offering protection against cellular damage and supporting overall health.

- Polyphenols:

 These are a type of antioxidant found in fruits like grapes, cherries, and apples.

 Polyphenols have been shown to improve insulin sensitivity and reduce inflammation, both of which are beneficial for managing diabetes.

- Flavonoids:

Found in abundance in berries, citrus fruits, and grapes, flavonoids are another group of antioxidants that have been linked to improved heart health and reduced risk of diabetes-related complications.

They help in reducing oxidative stress and inflammation, two key factors that can exacerbate diabetes.

Fiber: A Diabetic's Best Friend

One of the standout benefits of fruit for diabetics is its high fiber content.

Dietary fiber, particularly soluble fiber, plays a crucial role in controlling blood sugar levels.

When you eat fiber-rich fruits, the fiber slows down the digestion and absorption of sugars, which helps prevent sudden spikes in blood glucose levels.

- Soluble Fiber:

This type of fiber dissolves in water to form a gel-like substance in the digestive system.

It can slow down the absorption of glucose, making it particularly beneficial for diabetics.

Fruits like apples, oranges, and pears are excellent sources of soluble fiber.

- Insoluble Fiber:

 Although insoluble fiber does not have a direct impact on blood sugar levels, it is important for digestive health.

 It helps to prevent constipation, which is a common issue among diabetics, especially those who may have neuropathy affecting the gut.

 Insoluble fiber is found in the skins of fruits, such as apples and pears.

Low Glycemic Index (GI) Fruits

One of the key concepts for diabetics to understand is the glycemic index (GI), a scale that ranks carbohydrates on a scale from 0 to 100 based on how quickly and how much they raise blood sugar levels after eating.

Low-GI foods are those that score 55 or less, and they have a slower, smaller impact on blood glucose levels, making them ideal for diabetics.

The glycemic index is an important tool for diabetics because it helps predict how different foods will affect blood sugar levels.

Foods with a high GI are quickly digested and absorbed, causing rapid spikes in blood glucose, which can be particularly dangerous for diabetics.

On the other hand, low-GI foods are digested and absorbed more slowly, leading to a gradual rise in blood sugar levels.

- Why Low-GI Fruits are
Important:

 For diabetics, consuming low-
GI fruits means a more
controlled release of glucose
into the bloodstream, which can
help in maintaining stable blood
sugar levels throughout the day.

 This stability is crucial in
preventing both short-term
complications, such as
hyperglycemia, and long-term
complications, like nerve
damage and cardiovascular
disease.

Examples of Low-GI Fruits Beneficial for Diabetics

Here are some low-GI fruits that can be particularly beneficial for those managing diabetes:

- Apples:

With a GI score of around 39, apples are a great option for diabetics. They are rich in fiber, particularly pectin, which helps slow down the release of sugars into the bloodstream.

- Berries:

 Strawberries, blueberries, and raspberries all have a GI score of less than 40.

 They are packed with fiber and antioxidants, making them an excellent choice for managing blood sugar levels.

- Cherries:

 With a GI score of about 20, cherries are one of the best fruits for diabetics.

 They contain anthocyanins, which are antioxidants that help increase insulin production.

- Pears:

 Scoring around 38 on the GI scale, pears are rich in fiber and provide a satisfying sweetness without causing a significant spike in blood sugar levels.

- Peaches:

 With a GI of about 42, peaches are another good option.

 They are low in calories and high in fiber, making them a satisfying and diabetes-friendly fruit.

How to Incorporate Low-GI Fruits into a Diabetic-Friendly Diet

Including low-GI fruits in your diet is relatively simple and can be done in a variety of ways:

- As a Snack:

Enjoy an apple or a handful of berries as a mid-morning or afternoon snack.

Their natural sweetness can satisfy cravings while keeping blood sugar levels in check.

- In Salads:

 Add slices of pear or peaches to your salad for a refreshing and sweet contrast to greens and nuts. This not only enhances flavor but also adds fiber, which aids in digestion.

- In Smoothies:

 Create a diabetic-friendly smoothie by blending low-GI fruits like berries with unsweetened almond milk or yogurt. This makes for a filling and nutritious breakfast or snack.

- In Desserts:

  Use low-GI fruits in desserts, such as baked apples or a berry compote, to satisfy your sweet tooth without the need for added sugars.

Role of Phytochemicals in Fruits

 Phytochemicals are naturally occurring compounds in plants that have been found to provide various health benefits.

 In fruits, these compounds can have a significant impact on health, particularly for those with diabetes. Understanding the role of phytochemicals and how they can support diabetes management is crucial for anyone looking to optimize their diet.

Understanding Phytochemicals and Their Health Benefits

Phytochemicals are bioactive compounds found in fruits and vegetables that are not essential nutrients like vitamins and minerals but still provide significant health benefits.

They contribute to the color, flavor, and aroma of fruits, and many have powerful antioxidant properties.

- Types of Phytochemicals in Fruits:

- Flavonoids:

These include quercetin, kaempferol, and anthocyanins, which are found in berries, apples, and citrus fruits.

Flavonoids have anti-inflammatory and antioxidant properties, which can help reduce the risk of diabetes-related complications.

- Carotenoids:

 Found in fruits like papayas, mangoes, and apricots, carotenoids like beta-carotene have antioxidant properties and may improve insulin sensitivity.

- Phenolic Acids:

 Present in fruits like grapes, cherries, and apples, phenolic acids have been shown to help lower blood glucose levels and improve overall metabolic health.

Specific Fruits with High Levels of Beneficial Phytochemicals

 Certain fruits are particularly rich in phytochemicals that can offer specific benefits for diabetics:

- Blueberries:

 High in anthocyanins, blueberries have been shown to improve insulin sensitivity and lower the risk of type 2 diabetes. They are also rich in fiber, which aids in blood sugar regulation.

- Citrus Fruits:

 Oranges, lemons, and limes contain high levels of flavonoids, particularly hesperidin and naringenin, which have anti-inflammatory and blood sugar-lowering effects.

- Apples: Rich in quercetin, a flavonoid with anti-inflammatory properties, apples can help lower the risk of chronic diseases, including diabetes. Their high fiber content also helps in managing blood glucose levels.

- Grapes:

  Contain resveratrol, a type of polyphenol that has been shown to improve insulin sensitivity and protect against the oxidative stress that often accompanies diabetes.

Research Studies Supporting the Health Benefits of Fruits in Diabetes Management

Numerous studies have highlighted the positive effects of fruit consumption on diabetes management:

- The Nurses' Health Study:

This long-term study found that increased fruit consumption, particularly of berries, apples, and citrus fruits, was associated with a reduced risk of developing type 2 diabetes.

The high levels of antioxidants and fiber in these fruits are believed to contribute to their protective effects.

- Harvard School of Public Health Research:

 A study conducted by Harvard researchers found that individuals who ate at least two servings of whole fruits per day, especially blueberries, grapes, and apples, had a significantly lower risk of developing type 2 diabetes.

This study emphasized the importance of choosing whole fruits over fruit juices, which can cause rapid spikes in blood sugar.

- Journal of Nutrition Study:

A study published in the Journal of Nutrition found that flavonoid-rich fruits, such as berries, apples, and citrus fruits, were associated with a lower risk of insulin resistance and improved blood glucose control in individuals with type 2 diabetes.

<u>The Takeaway</u>

The nutritional benefits of fruit for diabetics cannot be overstated.

From vitamins and minerals that support overall health to fiber and phytochemicals that help manage blood sugar levels, fruits offer a wealth of benefits that can aid in diabetes management.

By making informed choices, such as selecting low-GI fruits and consuming them in moderation, diabetics can enjoy the sweetness and nutrition of fruit without compromising their health.

In the next chapter, we'll explore the "hate" side of the relationship between fruit and diabetes, delving into the challenges and potential risks of including fruit in a diabetic diet.

Chapter 2: The Hate – The Challenges of Including Fruit in a Diabetic Diet

High Sugar Content in Fruits

One of the primary concerns for diabetics when it comes to fruit is the natural sugar content.

While fruits are packed with essential nutrients, they also contain sugars that can raise blood glucose levels. For diabetics, managing blood sugar is a daily challenge, and consuming foods high in sugar can complicate this task.

Understanding Natural Sugars in Fruit

 Fruits contain three main types of natural sugars: glucose, fructose, and sucrose.

- Glucose:

 This is the simplest form of sugar and is directly absorbed into the bloodstream, leading to an immediate increase in blood sugar levels. While glucose is a necessary energy source for the body, it must be carefully managed in diabetics to prevent hyperglycemia.

- Fructose:

 Often referred to as fruit sugar, fructose is metabolized differently from glucose.

 It is processed in the liver, where it is either converted into glucose or stored as fat.

 Excessive fructose intake can lead to insulin resistance, which is a significant concern for diabetics.

- Sucrose:

 Also known as table sugar, sucrose is a combination of glucose and fructose.

 It is naturally present in fruits and breaks down into its component sugars during digestion.

 Sucrose can cause rapid spikes in blood sugar levels, which can be problematic for diabetics.

Comparing Fruit Sugar to Added Sugars

There's a key distinction between the natural sugars found in fruit and the added sugars present in many processed foods.

Natural sugars in fruit come with fiber, vitamins, and other beneficial compounds that help moderate their impact on blood glucose. In contrast, added sugars lack these beneficial components and can cause more significant spikes in blood sugar levels.

- Fiber's Role in Mitigating
Sugar Spikes:

 The fiber in fruit slows down
the absorption of sugar into the
bloodstream, helping to prevent
sharp spikes in blood glucose
levels.

 This is why whole fruits are
generally considered safer for
diabetics compared to fruit
juices or processed foods with
added sugars, which lack fiber
and can lead to rapid increases
in blood sugar.

- Portion Control and Sugar Intake:

 Even though the sugar in fruit is natural, portion control is essential for diabetics.

 Consuming large amounts of fruit can still lead to excessive sugar intake, which can be detrimental to blood sugar control.

 This is why understanding portion sizes and choosing fruits with lower sugar content is crucial.

High-Sugar Fruits to Be Cautious With

 While fruits like berries and apples have moderate sugar content, others are naturally higher in sugar and should be consumed in moderation by diabetics:

- Grapes:
 Grapes contain a significant amount of sugar, with a single cup providing about 23 grams. This can cause a rapid increase in blood glucose levels, particularly if consumed in large quantities.

- Mangoes:
 Known for their sweet, rich flavor, mangoes are high in sugar, with about 45 grams in a single fruit. This makes them a risky choice for diabetics, especially if consumed without considering portion sizes.

- Bananas:
 A medium banana contains about 14 grams of sugar. While bananas also provide fiber, their higher sugar content means they should be consumed with caution.

- Cherries:

 While cherries are low on the glycemic index, they are relatively high in sugar, with around 18 grams per cup.

 Diabetics need to monitor their intake to avoid potential blood sugar spikes.

<u>The Glycemic Load of Fruits</u>

In addition to considering the glycemic index (GI) of fruits, it's also important for diabetics to understand the concept of glycemic load (GL).

While the GI measures how quickly a food raises blood sugar levels, the GL takes into account the carbohydrate content of a standard serving of the food, providing a more comprehensive picture of its impact on blood glucose.

Differences Between Glycemic Index and Glycemic Load

- Glycemic Index (GI):

 As previously discussed, the GI ranks foods on a scale from 0 to 100 based on how quickly they raise blood sugar levels.

 Low-GI foods (55 or less) are digested more slowly, leading to a gradual increase in blood glucose.

- Glycemic Load (GL):

  The GL is calculated by multiplying the GI by the number of carbohydrates in a serving and then dividing by 100.

  This measure accounts for both the quality (GI) and quantity (carbohydrate content) of the carbohydrates in a food.

  A GL of 10 or less is considered low, while a GL of 20 or more is high.

  Understanding both GI and GL is important for diabetics because some fruits with a low GI might still have a high GL if consumed in large portions, leading to significant increases in blood sugar levels.

High Glycemic Load Fruits and Their Effects on Blood Sugar Spikes

Fruits with a high glycemic load can cause more pronounced spikes in blood glucose levels, making them less ideal for diabetics.

Here are a few examples:

- Watermelon:

 While watermelon has a low calorie count, its GI is quite high (about 72), and its GL can also be high if consumed in large quantities.

 A typical serving of watermelon (about 1 cup) has a GL of around 8, but larger portions can significantly increase this number, leading to a rapid rise in blood sugar.

- Pineapple:

 Pineapple has a moderate GI of around 66, but its high carbohydrate content gives it a higher GL, especially if consumed in large portions.

 A cup of pineapple chunks has a GL of about 6, but larger servings can push this number up, causing more noticeable blood sugar spikes.

- Ripe Bananas:

 As bananas ripen, their GI increases, and so does their GL.

 A medium ripe banana has a GI of around 51 and a GL of 10, making it a food that can lead to moderate increases in blood sugar levels, particularly if eaten in large quantities.

- Dates:

 Dates are extremely high in sugar, with a GI of around 103 and a very high GL, making them one of the riskiest fruits for diabetics.

 Even a small serving can cause significant spikes in blood glucose.

<u>Practical Examples of How Portion Sizes Can Affect Glycemic Load</u>

For diabetics, portion control is essential when consuming fruits, especially those with higher GIs and Gls.

Here's how portion sizes can affect the glycemic load of different fruits:

- Apples:

 A small apple (about 100 grams) has a GI of 39 and a GL of around 6.

 If you consume a large apple (about 223 grams), the GL increases to approximately 13, making it more likely to impact blood sugar levels significantly.

- Grapes:

 A small serving of grapes (about 50 grams) has a low GL of 3, but doubling the portion size to 100 grams raises the GL to 6.

 While the GI remains the same, the increased carbohydrate intake from the larger portion leads to a higher GL.

- Oranges:

 A medium orange (about 130 grams) has a GI of 40 and a GL of 5.5.

 If you eat two oranges, the GL doubles to 11, which can have a more substantial effect on blood sugar levels.

- Watermelon:

 A small serving of watermelon (about 120 grams) has a GL of around 5.

 If you consume 300 grams (equivalent to about 2 cups), the GL increases to 12.5, which can cause a noticeable spike in blood sugar.

Individual Responses to Fruit Consumption

Another challenge in managing diabetes is the fact that individuals respond differently to the same foods, including fruits.

While some diabetics may be able to enjoy certain fruits without significant blood sugar spikes, others may experience more pronounced effects. This variability makes it crucial for diabetics to monitor their blood sugar levels closely and adjust their diet accordingly.

Variation in Blood Sugar Responses Among Diabetics

 Several factors can influence how a diabetic's body responds to fruit consumption:

- Type of Diabetes:

 Individuals with type 1 diabetes may experience more dramatic blood sugar swings in response to certain fruits compared to those with type 2 diabetes, who may have more stable, albeit elevated, blood sugar levels.

- Insulin Sensitivity:

 People with higher insulin sensitivity may be able to process the sugars in fruit more effectively, leading to smaller increases in blood sugar levels.

 Those with insulin resistance, common in type 2 diabetes, may see higher spikes.

- Medication:

 The type and dosage of diabetes medication can also affect how the body handles the sugars in fruit.

 For example, individuals on insulin or insulin-stimulating medications might need to adjust their dosage based on their fruit intake to avoid hypoglycemia or hyperglycemia.

- Metabolism:

 Metabolic rates vary from person to person, affecting how quickly the body breaks down and absorbs the sugars in fruit.

 A faster metabolism might lead to quicker spikes in blood sugar, while a slower metabolism might result in a more gradual increase.

Factors That Influence These Responses

Beyond the individual factors, other aspects can influence how a diabetic responds to fruit consumption:

- Ripeness of the Fruit:

As fruits ripen, their sugar content increases, and so does their GI and GL. For example, a ripe banana has a higher sugar content and a higher GI than a green banana, leading to a more significant impact on blood sugar levels.

- Combination with Other Foods:

 Eating fruit alongside other foods, particularly those rich in protein or fat, can slow down the absorption of sugars and reduce the overall impact on blood sugar levels.

 For example, pairing apple slices with peanut butter can help moderate the blood sugar response.

- Time of Day:

  Blood sugar levels can fluctuate throughout the day due to hormonal changes, physical activity, and meal timing.

  Some diabetics may find that they tolerate fruit better at certain times of the day, such as in the morning or after a workout, when their insulin sensitivity is higher.

The Importance of Self-Monitoring and Individualized Dietary Plans

Given the variability in how diabetics respond to fruit, self-monitoring is essential.

Diabetics should regularly check their blood sugar levels before and after consuming fruit to understand how it affects them personally. This information can then be used to create an individualized dietary plan that balances the enjoyment of fruit with the need for blood sugar control.

- Using a Glucometer:

 Regularly using a glucometer to monitor blood sugar levels can help diabetics track how different fruits affect them.

 Keeping a food diary alongside blood sugar readings can reveal patterns and help identify which fruits are better tolerated.

- Consulting a Dietitian:

 Working with a registered
dietitian or diabetes educator
can help diabetics create a
personalized eating plan that
includes fruits while minimizing
the risk of blood sugar spikes.

 A dietitian can provide
guidance on portion sizes, fruit
combinations, and meal timing
to optimize blood sugar control.

- Experimenting with Timing and Combinations:

 Diabetics can experiment with different times of day and food combinations to see what works best for them.

 For example, some may find that they tolerate fruit better when consumed as part of a balanced meal rather than on its own.

<u>The Takeaway</u>

While fruits offer numerous health benefits, they also present unique challenges for diabetics.

High sugar content, the glycemic load of certain fruits, and individual variability in blood sugar responses can make fruit consumption a tricky area to navigate. However, with careful monitoring, portion control, and individualized dietary planning, diabetics can enjoy the nutritional benefits of fruit without compromising their blood sugar control.

In the next chapter, we'll focus on practical strategies for navigating this love-hate relationship, including smart fruit choices, timing, and recipes that make fruit a healthy part of a diabetic diet.

Chapter 3: Navigating the Love-Hate Relationship**

Smart Fruit Choices for Diabetics

For diabetics, making informed decisions about which fruits to include in their diet is key to balancing the nutritional benefits with blood sugar control.

By choosing fruits that are lower in sugar and higher in fiber, diabetics can enjoy the health benefits of fruit without experiencing significant spikes in blood sugar levels.

List of Fruits to Enjoy

 Certain fruits are more suitable for diabetics due to their lower glycemic index, higher fiber content, and lower sugar levels.

 Here's a list of fruits that diabetics can enjoy in moderation:

- Berries:

 Strawberries, blueberries, raspberries, and blackberries are all excellent choices.

 They are low in sugar, high in fiber, and packed with antioxidants.

 Berries have a low glycemic index, typically ranging from 25 to 40, making them a smart choice for managing blood sugar levels.

- Apples:

 Apples are rich in fiber, particularly in the skin, and have a glycemic index of around 39.

 They provide a slow release of sugar into the bloodstream, which helps prevent spikes in blood sugar.

- Pears:

  Similar to apples, pears are high in fiber and have a low glycemic index (around 38).

  They are also a good source of vitamins and minerals, making them a healthy option for diabetics.

- Cherries:

 With a low glycemic index of about 22, cherries are another great fruit for diabetics.

 They contain anthocyanins, which may help lower blood sugar levels and reduce inflammation.

- Citrus Fruits:

 Oranges, grapefruits, and lemons are all low-GI fruits, with glycemic indexes ranging from 31 to 51.

 They are high in vitamin C and fiber, making them beneficial for overall health and blood sugar control.

- Peaches:

 Peaches have a glycemic index of around 42 and are low in calories.

 They are also high in fiber and vitamins, making them a good choice for a diabetes-friendly diet.

- Avocados:

 Although technically a fruit, avocados are unique in that they are low in carbohydrates and have almost no sugar.

 They are rich in healthy fats and fiber, which can help manage blood sugar levels and improve insulin sensitivity.

Fruits to Avoid or Limit

While many fruits can be enjoyed in moderation, some are higher in sugar and have a higher glycemic index, making them less ideal for diabetics.

Here are some fruits that should be consumed sparingly:

- Mangoes:

 Mangoes are delicious but high in sugar, with a glycemic index of around 51.

 A single mango can contain over 45 grams of sugar, which can lead to significant spikes in blood glucose levels.

- Bananas:

 Bananas, particularly ripe ones, have a higher glycemic index (around 51) and are relatively high in sugar.

 Diabetics should consider eating them in small portions and pairing them with protein or fat to slow down sugar absorption.

- Grapes:

 Grapes have a glycemic index
of about 59 and are high in
sugar, with a single cup
containing around 23 grams.

 Eating them in large quantities
can lead to rapid increases in
blood sugar.

- Pineapple:

 Pineapple has a glycemic index of around 66, making it a high-GI fruit.

 It is also high in sugar, so it should be consumed in small portions.

- Watermelon:

 Watermelon has a glycemic index of about 72, which is quite high.

 While it is low in calories, its high GI and high sugar content make it a fruit that should be limited in a diabetic diet.

How to Pair Fruits with Other Foods to Minimize Blood Sugar Spikes

 Combining fruits with other foods, particularly those high in protein or healthy fats, can help slow down the digestion and absorption of sugar, reducing the impact on blood glucose levels.

 Here are some tips for pairing fruits with other foods:

- Add Nuts or Seeds:

  Pairing fruits like apples, pears, or berries with a handful of nuts (e.g., almonds, walnuts) or seeds (e.g., chia, flaxseeds) can add healthy fats and protein, which help slow down the sugar absorption process.

- Combine with Dairy:

  Eating fruits with Greek yogurt or cottage cheese provides protein and fat, which can help stabilize blood sugar levels.

  For example, a bowl of berries with a dollop of Greek yogurt makes a satisfying and blood sugar-friendly snack.

- Include Whole Grains:

 Pairing fruits with whole grains, such as oatmeal or whole-grain bread, adds fiber and protein, helping to prevent blood sugar spikes.

 For instance, topping oatmeal with sliced apples or berries can create a balanced and filling breakfast.

- Use Avocado:

 Avocados are rich in healthy fats and can be paired with fruits like strawberries or oranges to create a refreshing and blood sugar-friendly salad.

 The fat in avocados helps slow down the digestion of sugars in the fruit.

- Incorporate Nut Butters:

 Spreading almond or peanut butter on apple slices or pairing banana slices with nut butter on whole-grain toast can add protein and fat, making the fruit more diabetes-friendly.

Timing and Frequency of Fruit Consumption

 When and how often you eat fruit can significantly affect blood sugar levels.

 Timing fruit consumption strategically throughout the day can help diabetics enjoy the benefits of fruit without experiencing unwanted blood sugar spikes.

<u>Best Times to Eat Fruit for Optimal Blood Sugar Control</u>

- In the Morning:

  Eating fruit in the morning, as part of a balanced breakfast, can provide a natural source of energy and fiber to start the day.

  Combining fruit with protein and healthy fats, such as eggs, yogurt, or avocado, can help maintain stable blood sugar levels throughout the morning.

- Before or After Exercise:

 Consuming fruit before or after exercise can be beneficial for diabetics.

 Before exercise, fruit provides a quick source of energy, while after exercise, it helps replenish glycogen stores.

 Pairing fruit with protein, such as a handful of nuts or a protein shake, can further stabilize blood sugar levels.

- As a Mid-Morning or
Afternoon Snack:

 Including fruit as a snack
between meals can help prevent
blood sugar dips and keep
energy levels steady.

 Pairing fruit with protein or fat
can help avoid spikes in blood
glucose.

- In the Evening:

 While some diabetics may worry about eating fruit in the evening, it can still be a part of a balanced diet if consumed in moderation and paired with protein or healthy fats.

 For example, a small bowl of berries with Greek yogurt can be a light and satisfying evening snack.

How Often Diabetics Should Include Fruit in Their Diet

The frequency of fruit consumption depends on individual blood sugar control, dietary preferences, and overall health.

However, here are some general guidelines for diabetics:

- Moderation is Key:

 Diabetics can enjoy fruit daily, but moderation is crucial.

 Including one to three servings of fruit per day, spread out across meals and snacks, is generally a safe approach.

 It's important to monitor blood sugar levels to determine the right amount and frequency.

- Spreading Fruit Intake Throughout the Day:

 Rather than consuming large amounts of fruit in one sitting, spreading fruit intake throughout the day can help maintain stable blood sugar levels.

 For example, a serving of fruit with breakfast, another as a snack, and a small portion with dinner can provide balanced nutrition without causing significant blood sugar fluctuations.

- Incorporating a Variety of Fruits:

 Including a variety of fruits in your diet ensures that you receive a broad spectrum of nutrients.

 Rotating different types of low-GI fruits can help prevent boredom and provide a range of vitamins, minerals, and antioxidants.

- Monitoring Blood Sugar
Levels:

 Regularly checking blood sugar
levels after consuming fruit can
help diabetics understand how
different fruits affect them.

 This information can guide
decisions about how often to
include fruit in their diet and in
what portions.

Diabetes-Friendly Fruit Recipes

Incorporating fruit into a diabetic-friendly diet doesn't have to be difficult.

With the right recipes and preparation methods, diabetics can enjoy fruit in delicious and satisfying ways that support blood sugar control.

<u>Smoothies</u>

Smoothies are a versatile and easy way to include fruit in your diet.

By using low-GI fruits and adding protein and healthy fats, you can create a balanced, diabetes-friendly smoothie.

Berry Avocado Smoothie

- Ingredients:

  - 1/2 avocado
  - 1/2 cup frozen blueberries
  - 1/2 cup frozen strawberries
  - 1/2 cup unsweetened almond
milk
  - 1/4 cup Greek yogurt
  - 1 tablespoon chia seeds
  - 1/2 cup water (optional, for
thinning)

- Instructions:

1. Combine all ingredients in a blender.
2. Blend until smooth, adding water if needed to reach your desired consistency.
3. Serve immediately and enjoy a creamy, nutritious smoothie that's low in sugar and high in fiber.

Apple Cinnamon Protein Smoothie

- Ingredients:

  - 1 small apple, cored and chopped
  - 1/2 banana (preferably green or less ripe)
  - 1 scoop vanilla protein powder
  - 1/2 teaspoon ground cinnamon
  - 1/2 cup unsweetened almond milk
  - 1/2 cup water or ice

- Instructions:

1. Add all ingredients to a blender.
2. Blend until smooth.
3. Pour into a glass and enjoy a protein-packed smoothie that's perfect for breakfast or a post-workout snack.

Salads

Fruit can add a burst of flavor and color to salads, making them more enjoyable and nutritious.

Here's a diabetes-friendly salad recipe that combines fruit with greens, nuts, and a light dressing.

Spinach and Berry Salad

- Ingredients:

  - 2 cups fresh spinach leaves
  - 1/2 cup sliced strawberries
  - 1/4 cup blueberries
  - 1/4 cup crumbled feta cheese
  - 1/4 cup chopped walnuts
  - 1 tablespoon balsamic
vinegar
  - 1 tablespoon olive oil
  - Salt and pepper to taste

- Instructions:

1. In a large bowl, combine spinach, strawberries, blueberries, feta cheese, and walnuts.
2. In a small bowl, whisk together balsamic vinegar, olive oil, salt, and pepper.
3. Drizzle the dressing over the salad and toss to combine.
4. Serve immediately as a refreshing and nutritious meal or side dish.

Citrus Avocado Salad

- Ingredients:

  - 1 orange, peeled and segmented
  - 1/2 grapefruit, peeled and segmented
  - 1 avocado, sliced
  - 2 cups mixed greens (e.g., arugula, spinach, kale)
  - 1 tablespoon olive oil
  - 1 tablespoon lemon juice
  - 1 teaspoon honey (optional, or substitute with a non-sugar sweetener)
  - Salt and pepper to taste

- Instructions:

1. In a large bowl, combine mixed greens, orange segments, grapefruit segments, and avocado slices.
2. In a small bowl, whisk together olive oil, lemon juice, honey, salt, and pepper.
3. Drizzle the dressing over the salad and toss gently to combine.
4. Serve as a light and refreshing dish that balances sweet and savory flavors.

Desserts

Creating diabetes-friendly desserts doesn't mean you have to sacrifice flavor.

By choosing low-GI fruits and using alternative sweeteners, you can enjoy satisfying sweets without spiking your blood sugar.

Baked Apples with Cinnamon

- Ingredients:

  - 2 medium apples, cored and sliced
  - 1/2 teaspoon ground cinnamon
  - 1 tablespoon chopped nuts (e.g., walnuts, pecans)
  - 1 tablespoon unsweetened coconut flakes (optional)
  - 1 teaspoon butter or coconut oil

- Instructions:

1. Preheat the oven to 350°F (175°C).
2. Place apple slices in a baking dish.
3. Sprinkle with cinnamon, nuts, and coconut flakes.
4. Dot with butter or coconut oil.
5. Bake for 20-25 minutes until apples are tender.
6. Serve warm, optionally with a dollop of Greek yogurt.

Berry Yogurt Parfait

- Ingredients:

  - 1/2 cup Greek yogurt
  - 1/4 cup mixed berries (e.g., blueberries, strawberries, raspberries)
  - 1 tablespoon chopped nuts or seeds
  - 1 teaspoon honey or sugar-free sweetener (optional)

- Instructions:

1. In a small glass or bowl, layer half of the yogurt, followed by half of the berries.
2. Repeat the layers with the remaining yogurt and berries.
3. Top with chopped nuts or seeds and a drizzle of honey, if desired.
4. Serve as a quick and healthy dessert or snack.

The Takeaway

Navigating the love-hate relationship between fruit and diabetes requires knowledge, careful planning, and a bit of creativity in the kitchen.

By choosing the right fruits, pairing them with complementary foods, and timing their consumption strategically, diabetics can enjoy the many health benefits of fruit while maintaining stable blood sugar levels.

With the help of diabetes-friendly recipes, fruit can be a delicious and nutritious part of a balanced diet.

In the next chapter, we'll explore the emotional and psychological aspects of this relationship, discussing the challenges of food restrictions and strategies for maintaining a positive relationship with food while managing diabetes.

Chapter 4: The Emotional and Psychological Aspects

The Psychological Impact of Food Restrictions

 For many diabetics, managing the condition involves a constant battle with food restrictions.

 These restrictions, while necessary for maintaining health, can have significant emotional and psychological effects.

Fruit, often considered a symbol of health and vitality, can become a source of anxiety and frustration when it must be limited or avoided due to diabetes.

Emotional Challenges of Managing Diabetes

The emotional challenges that come with managing diabetes are often underestimated.

For many diabetics, the need to constantly monitor and regulate food intake can lead to feelings of deprivation, guilt, and even resentment.

The relationship with food, which should be nourishing and enjoyable, can become fraught with stress and anxiety.

- Feelings of Deprivation:

 Being told to limit or avoid certain foods, especially those that are generally considered healthy, like fruit, can lead to a sense of deprivation.

 This is particularly challenging when these foods are ones that the individual enjoys or associates with positive experiences, such as family gatherings, holidays, or cultural traditions.

- Guilt and Anxiety:

 Many diabetics experience guilt or anxiety around food, especially when they indulge in something that might not align with their dietary restrictions.

 This can create a negative cycle where food choices are driven by guilt rather than enjoyment, further complicating the relationship with food.

- Social and Cultural Pressures:

 Food is often at the center of social gatherings and cultural events.

 Diabetics may feel isolated or different when they have to turn down certain foods or bring their own diabetic-friendly options to events.

 This can lead to feelings of exclusion or frustration, especially if others don't understand the seriousness of their dietary needs.

- The Pressure of Perfection:

 Many diabetics feel immense pressure to "get it right" with their diet, which can lead to stress and anxiety.

 The fear of making a mistake and the potential consequences for their health can be overwhelming, making it difficult to enjoy food without constant worry.

The Psychological Effect of Being Told to Limit or Avoid Certain Fruits

Fruit, with its natural sweetness and nutritional benefits, is often seen as a healthy and positive food choice.

Being told to limit or avoid certain fruits because of diabetes can be particularly disheartening, as it challenges the commonly held belief that "all fruits are good for you."

- Mixed Messages:

 Diabetics often receive mixed messages about fruit.

 On one hand, fruits are promoted as healthy, nutrient-dense foods that should be part of a balanced diet.

 On the other hand, diabetics are warned about the sugar content in fruits and the potential impact on blood glucose levels. This conflicting information can lead to confusion and frustration, making it difficult to make informed decisions.

- Cravings and Temptations:

 Being told to limit or avoid certain fruits can also intensify cravings for those very foods.

 This is a common psychological response to restriction, where the more something is off-limits, the more it is desired.

 For diabetics, this can create a difficult internal struggle between wanting to enjoy fruit and needing to manage blood sugar levels.

- Loss of Food Enjoyment:

 For many people, fruit is a source of enjoyment and satisfaction, providing a sweet treat that feels both indulgent and healthy.

 When diabetics are told to limit or avoid fruit, it can lead to a loss of enjoyment in their diet, making meals and snacks feel less satisfying and more like a chore.

Coping Strategies for Dealing with Cravings and Food Restrictions

Managing cravings and dealing with food restrictions is a significant aspect of living with diabetes.

However, there are several strategies that can help diabetics cope with these challenges and maintain a positive relationship with food.

- Mindful Eating:

 Practicing mindful eating involves being fully present during meals and snacks, paying attention to the taste, texture, and satisfaction derived from each bite.

 This approach can help diabetics enjoy their food more fully and reduce the urge to overindulge in restricted foods. By savoring each bite of a small portion of fruit, for example, diabetics can satisfy their cravings without compromising their blood sugar control.

- Finding Healthy Substitutes:

 When certain fruits are off-limits or need to be limited, finding healthy substitutes can help satisfy cravings.

 For example, if mangoes are too high in sugar, diabetics can try a lower-sugar fruit like berries or a sugar-free fruit-flavored dessert that mimics the taste without the glucose spike.

- Portion Control:

 Instead of completely avoiding certain fruits, diabetics can focus on portion control to manage their intake.

 Having a small portion of a higher-sugar fruit occasionally can satisfy a craving without causing significant harm to blood sugar levels.

 This approach allows diabetics to enjoy a variety of fruits without feeling deprived.

- Incorporating Fruits into Balanced Meals:

 Including fruit as part of a balanced meal, rather than eating it alone, can help mitigate its impact on blood sugar levels.

 Pairing fruit with protein or fat, as discussed in the previous chapter, can slow down the absorption of sugar and provide a more satisfying eating experience.

- Seeking Support:

 Talking to a dietitian, diabetes educator, or support group can provide diabetics with the tools and encouragement they need to manage cravings and food restrictions.

 Sharing experiences with others who understand the challenges of living with diabetes can help reduce feelings of isolation and frustration.

Balancing Enjoyment and Health

One of the most important aspects of managing diabetes is finding a balance between enjoying food and maintaining good health.

While it's essential to make choices that support blood sugar control, it's equally important to enjoy what you eat.
A diet that feels restrictive or joyless is difficult to sustain, which can lead to burnout and poor management of the condition.

The Importance of Finding Pleasure in Food While Managing Diabetes

Food is more than just fuel for the body; it's a source of pleasure, comfort, and connection.

For diabetics, finding ways to enjoy food while managing blood sugar levels is crucial for long-term success in managing the condition.

- Creating Satisfying Meals:

 By focusing on the flavors, textures, and colors of food, diabetics can create meals that are both satisfying and healthy.

 This might involve experimenting with new recipes, trying different fruits and vegetables, or incorporating herbs and spices to enhance flavor without adding sugar or salt.

- Allowing for Occasional
Indulgences:

 It's important for diabetics to
allow themselves occasional
indulgences.

 Completely eliminating favorite
foods can lead to feelings of
deprivation and increase the risk
of binge eating.

 By planning for small,
controlled indulgences, diabetics
can enjoy their favorite foods
without derailing their blood
sugar control.

- Prioritizing Quality Over Quantity:

 Instead of focusing on the quantity of food, diabetics can prioritize the quality of their meals.

 Choosing fresh, whole ingredients and savoring smaller portions of high-quality foods can lead to a more satisfying eating experience.

- Practicing Gratitude:

 Taking a moment to express gratitude for the food you're about to eat can shift your focus from what you can't have to what you can enjoy.

 This practice can enhance the overall eating experience and help diabetics appreciate the nourishing foods they can include in their diet.

Tips for Satisfying Sweet Cravings Without Overindulging in High-Sugar Fruits

Managing sweet cravings is a common challenge for diabetics, especially when trying to limit high-sugar fruits.

Here are some strategies to satisfy those cravings without compromising blood sugar control:

- Choose Low-GI Fruits:

 As mentioned in previous chapters, choosing low-GI fruits like berries, apples, and pears can provide sweetness without causing significant spikes in blood sugar.

 These fruits can be enjoyed on their own or incorporated into desserts and snacks.

- Use Natural Sweeteners:

  Natural, low-calorie sweeteners like stevia or monk fruit can be used to sweeten dishes without adding sugar.

  These sweeteners can be added to Greek yogurt, smoothies, or baked goods to create satisfying, diabetes-friendly treats.

- Opt for Frozen or Dried Fruit:

  Frozen or dried fruit can be a convenient and satisfying way to satisfy sweet cravings.

  However, it's important to choose unsweetened varieties and to watch portion sizes, as dried fruit is more concentrated in sugar and calories.

- Incorporate Cinnamon and Spices:

 Adding cinnamon, nutmeg, or other spices to dishes can enhance the natural sweetness of fruits and reduce the need for added sugar.

 For example, sprinkling cinnamon on baked apples or pears can create a warm, comforting dessert with minimal impact on blood sugar.

- Make Fruit-Based Desserts:

 Creating desserts that feature fruit as the main ingredient can satisfy sweet cravings while providing the nutritional benefits of fruit.

 Recipes like baked apples, berry parfaits, or fruit salads can be delicious and diabetes-friendly options.

Encouraging a Positive Relationship with Food, Including Fruit

 Fostering a positive relationship with food is essential for diabetics to maintain a healthy and balanced diet.

 This involves shifting the focus from what foods are off-limits to finding joy in the foods that support health and well-being.

- Reframe Your Mindset:

 Instead of viewing food restrictions as a burden, try to reframe your mindset to see them as opportunities to explore new foods and flavors.

 This positive outlook can help reduce feelings of deprivation and make it easier to stick to a healthy eating plan.

- Practice Self-Compassion:

 It's important for diabetics to be kind to themselves when it comes to food choices.

 Perfection is not the goal, and it's normal to have occasional indulgences or make mistakes.

 Practicing self-compassion can help reduce feelings of guilt and encourage a healthier relationship with food.

- Focus on Health Benefits:

  Reminding yourself of the health benefits of your food choices can help reinforce positive eating habits.

  For example, when choosing a low-GI fruit like berries, focus on the antioxidants, vitamins, and fiber you're getting, rather than on the sugar you're avoiding.

- Celebrate Small Wins:

 Acknowledge and celebrate the small successes in your diabetes management journey.

 Whether it's finding a new fruit you enjoy, successfully managing a craving, or maintaining stable blood sugar levels, celebrating these wins can boost motivation and reinforce healthy habits.

- Seek Joy in the Eating
Experience:

 Finally, take the time to enjoy
the overall eating experience.

 This includes the preparation,
presentation, and consumption
of your meals.

 Eating mindfully and
appreciating the sensory aspects
of food can enhance satisfaction
and reduce the desire to overeat
or indulge in less healthy
options.

<u>**The Takeaway**</u>

The emotional and psychological aspects of managing diabetes are just as important as the physical aspects.

By finding ways to balance enjoyment and health, diabetics can maintain a positive relationship with food and avoid the pitfalls of deprivation and guilt.

Mindful eating, portion control, and allowing for occasional indulgences can help diabetics enjoy fruit and other foods as part of a healthy, balanced diet.

In the next chapter, we'll explore the future of fruit in diabetic diets, looking at emerging research, the role of technology, and the importance of continued education in managing diabetes.

Chapter 5: The Future of Fruit in Diabetic Diets

Emerging Research on Fruit and Diabetes

As our understanding of diabetes and nutrition continues to evolve, so too does the research surrounding the role of fruit in a diabetic diet.

While the traditional approach has often been cautious, focusing on limiting high-sugar fruits, emerging studies are beginning to paint a more nuanced picture.

Researchers are now exploring the potential benefits of certain fruits, the role of bioactive compounds, and how personalized nutrition might change the way diabetics approach their diet.

New Studies and Findings on the Benefits and Risks of Fruit for Diabetics

Recent research has begun to challenge the notion that all fruits should be limited in a diabetic diet.

Some studies suggest that certain fruits may offer protective benefits against diabetes and its complications, while others continue to highlight the risks associated with high sugar consumption.

- Protective Role of Berries:

 A study published in the American Journal of Clinical Nutrition found that regular consumption of berries, particularly blueberries, strawberries, and blackberries, is associated with a reduced risk of developing type 2 diabetes.

 The high levels of anthocyanins and other polyphenols in berries are thought to improve insulin sensitivity and reduce inflammation, which are key factors in diabetes management.

- Glycemic Response to Whole Fruit vs. Fruit Juices:

 Another important finding is the difference in glycemic response between whole fruits and fruit juices.

 Research published in the BMJ indicates that while whole fruits, particularly those high in fiber like apples and oranges, are associated with a lower risk of type 2 diabetes, fruit juices can have the opposite effect, increasing the risk due to their higher glycemic load and lack of fiber.

- Role of Fiber in Modulating Blood Sugar:

 A growing body of research highlights the importance of dietary fiber in managing diabetes.

 Studies have shown that high-fiber fruits, such as pears, apples, and berries, can help improve blood sugar control by slowing the absorption of glucose.
 This has led to a greater emphasis on promoting fiber-rich fruits as part of a diabetic diet.

- Potential Risks of Excess Fructose:

 Despite the benefits, there are still concerns about the fructose content in some fruits.

 Excessive fructose intake has been linked to insulin resistance, fatty liver disease, and increased visceral fat, which are all risk factors for type 2 diabetes.

 This has led researchers to recommend moderation, particularly with high-fructose fruits like mangoes and grapes.

- Bioactive Compounds in Fruit:

 Beyond their fiber and vitamin content, fruits contain various bioactive compounds that may have health benefits for diabetics.

 For example, flavonoids, found in abundance in berries and citrus fruits, have been shown to improve endothelial function and reduce oxidative stress, both of which are important for preventing diabetes-related complications.

Potential Future Recommendations for Fruit Consumption in Diabetes Management

Given the emerging research, future dietary recommendations for diabetics may become more individualized and nuanced.

Rather than broad restrictions on fruit, the focus may shift towards encouraging the consumption of specific fruits that offer health benefits while advising moderation on others.

- Personalized Nutrition:

 As the field of personalized nutrition grows, future guidelines may take into account an individual's genetic makeup, microbiome, and metabolic response to different foods.

 This could lead to more tailored recommendations for fruit consumption, allowing diabetics to enjoy a wider variety of fruits without compromising their blood sugar control.

- Emphasis on Whole Fruits:

 Future dietary guidelines are likely to continue emphasizing the importance of whole fruits over fruit juices.

 The benefits of fiber, along with the slower release of sugars into the bloodstream, make whole fruits a preferable choice for diabetics.

 Additionally, recommendations may focus on integrating fruit into meals rather than consuming it alone to further mitigate glycemic responses.

- Moderation and Variety:

 Rather than categorically avoiding certain fruits, future guidelines may emphasize moderation and variety.

 By encouraging diabetics to eat a wide range of low-GI fruits in appropriate portions, the aim will be to maximize nutritional benefits while minimizing blood sugar fluctuations.

- Education on Portion Sizes and Pairing:

 As part of future recommendations, there may be more emphasis on educating diabetics about portion sizes and the benefits of pairing fruits with protein, fat, or fiber-rich foods.

 This approach could help diabetics enjoy a broader spectrum of fruits while maintaining better blood sugar control.

The Evolving Understanding of Fruit's Role in a Diabetic Diet

As research continues to evolve, our understanding of fruit's role in a diabetic diet is likely to become more sophisticated.

The growing recognition of the importance of fiber, the potential benefits of certain bioactive compounds, and the impact of individual variation all point to a future where fruit can be enjoyed as part of a balanced, diabetes-friendly diet.

- Shifting Perspectives:

 The traditional view of fruit as a potential risk for diabetics due to its sugar content is gradually being challenged.

 As more research highlights the benefits of certain fruits, particularly those rich in fiber and antioxidants, there may be a shift towards a more balanced approach that considers both the benefits and the risks.

- Integration into Overall Diet:

 Rather than viewing fruit in isolation, future dietary guidelines may place greater emphasis on how fruit fits into the overall diet.

 This holistic approach considers the balance of macronutrients, the timing of fruit consumption, and the combination with other foods to optimize blood sugar control.

- Focus on Long-Term Health Outcomes:

As research continues to explore the long-term health outcomes associated with fruit consumption in diabetics, future guidelines may be shaped by a greater understanding of how specific fruits impact not just blood sugar, but also cardiovascular health, weight management, and overall well-being.

The Role of Technology in Managing Fruit Intake

Technology is playing an increasingly important role in diabetes management, offering tools and resources that can help diabetics make more informed dietary choices, including decisions about fruit intake.

From apps that track blood sugar levels to continuous glucose monitors (CGMs) that provide real-time data, technology is transforming the way diabetics manage their condition.

Use of Apps and Devices to Track Blood Sugar and Fruit Consumption

With the advent of smartphone apps and wearable devices, diabetics now have access to a wealth of information at their fingertips.

These tools can help diabetics monitor their blood sugar levels, track their food intake, and make more informed decisions about what they eat, including fruit.

- Food Tracking Apps:

 Apps like MyFitnessPal, Carb Manager, and Glucose Buddy allow users to log their meals and snacks, including fruit, and track their carbohydrate intake.

 Many of these apps also provide nutritional information, including glycemic index and load, which can help diabetics choose the right fruits and portion sizes.

- Blood Sugar Monitoring:

 Continuous glucose monitors (CGMs) like Dexcom and FreeStyle Libre provide real-time data on blood sugar levels, allowing diabetics to see how their body responds to different foods, including fruit.

 This information can help diabetics make more informed decisions about which fruits to include in their diet and how to pair them with other foods to minimize blood sugar spikes.

- Personalized
Recommendations:

 Some apps and devices are now offering personalized dietary recommendations based on an individual's blood sugar data.

 For example, after tracking blood sugar responses to different fruits, an app might suggest which fruits to eat more of and which to avoid, based on how they affect blood glucose levels.

- Meal Planning Tools:

 Technology is also making it easier for diabetics to plan their meals, including fruit.

 Apps that offer meal planning and recipe suggestions tailored to blood sugar goals can help diabetics integrate fruit into their diet in a balanced and controlled way.

How Technology Can Help Diabetics Make Informed Choices About Fruit

Technology is empowering diabetics to take control of their health by providing the data and tools they need to make informed dietary choices.

This is particularly important when it comes to managing fruit intake, as the impact of fruit on blood sugar can vary widely from person to person.

- Data-Driven Decisions:

 By using technology to track blood sugar levels and food intake, diabetics can make data-driven decisions about their diet.

 For example, if a diabetic notices that their blood sugar spikes after eating a certain fruit, they can use that information to adjust their portion size or pair it with other foods to reduce the impact.

- Real-Time Feedback:

 Continuous glucose monitors provide real-time feedback, allowing diabetics to see the immediate effects of their food choices.

 This can be particularly useful for managing fruit intake, as it allows diabetics to experiment with different fruits, portion sizes, and food combinations to see what works best for them.

- Increased Awareness and Education:

 Technology is also helping to increase awareness and education about the role of fruit in a diabetic diet.

 Many apps offer educational resources, articles, and tips on how to manage diabetes, including how to make smart fruit choices.

 This information can help diabetics feel more confident and empowered in their food choices.

- Support and Community:

 In addition to tracking and monitoring tools, many apps and devices offer access to online communities where diabetics can share experiences, tips, and advice about managing their condition, including how to navigate the challenges of fruit consumption.

 This sense of support and community can be invaluable in helping diabetics stay motivated and on track.

The Future of Personalized Nutrition and Its Implications for Diabetic Diets

As technology continues to advance, the future of personalized nutrition looks promising, particularly for diabetics. Personalized nutrition involves tailoring dietary recommendations to an individual's unique genetic makeup, microbiome, lifestyle, and health goals. This approach has the potential to revolutionize the way diabetics manage their diet, including how they approach fruit consumption.

- Genetic Testing:

 Genetic testing can provide insights into how an individual's body metabolizes different nutrients, including sugars.

 This information can be used to create personalized dietary plans that optimize blood sugar control while allowing for a more flexible and enjoyable diet, including the incorporation of fruit.

- Microbiome Analysis:

 The gut microbiome plays a crucial role in metabolism and blood sugar regulation.

 By analyzing an individual's microbiome, personalized nutrition plans can be developed that support a healthy gut and improve blood sugar control.

 This could lead to more tailored recommendations about which fruits are most beneficial for each individual.

- Artificial Intelligence (AI) and Machine Learning:

AI and machine learning are increasingly being used to analyze large amounts of health data and provide personalized dietary recommendations.

For diabetics, this could mean more precise guidance on which fruits to eat, when to eat them, and how to pair them with other foods to optimize blood sugar control.

- Integration with Wearable
Devices:

 The integration of personalized
nutrition with wearable devices
like CGMs and fitness trackers
is likely to become more
common.

 This will allow diabetics to
receive real-time, personalized
recommendations based on their
current blood sugar levels,
physical activity, and other
factors, making it easier to
manage their diet and health.

The Importance of Continued Education

As diabetes management continues to evolve, staying informed about the latest research, dietary guidelines, and technological advancements is crucial.

Continued education is essential for diabetics to make the best choices for their health, including how to incorporate fruit into their diet in a way that supports blood sugar control.

Why Staying Informed About Diabetes and Diet Is Crucial

Diabetes is a complex and evolving condition, and what we know about managing it continues to change as new research emerges.

For diabetics, staying informed about the latest developments in diet and nutrition is critical to making the best choices for their health.

- Adapting to New Research:

As new studies reveal more about the impact of fruit on blood sugar and overall health, diabetics may need to adjust their diet to align with the latest evidence.

Staying informed allows diabetics to make these adjustments proactively rather than relying on outdated information.

- Understanding Emerging Technologies:

 As technology plays an increasingly important role in diabetes management, understanding how to use new tools and devices is essential.

 Continued education can help diabetics make the most of these advancements and integrate them into their daily routine effectively.

- Navigating Conflicting Information:

 With so much information available online, it's important for diabetics to be able to discern credible sources from misinformation.

 Continued education can help diabetics navigate conflicting information and make informed decisions about their diet and health.

- Empowering Self-
Management:

The more informed diabetics
are about their condition, the
more empowered they are to
manage it effectively.

Continued education provides
diabetics with the knowledge
and tools they need to take
control of their health and make
choices that support their well-
being.

Resources for Diabetics to Keep Up with the Latest Information on Fruit and Diabetes

There are many resources available to help diabetics stay informed about the latest research and guidelines on fruit and diabetes.

These resources include:

- Diabetes Organizations:

 Organizations like the American Diabetes Association (ADA), Diabetes UK, and the International Diabetes Federation (IDF) provide up-to-date information on diabetes management, including dietary guidelines and the latest research on fruit and other foods.

- Scientific Journals:

For those interested in more in-depth information, scientific journals like Diabetes Care, The Lancet Diabetes & Endocrinology, and The Journal of Nutrition publish the latest research on diabetes and diet.

- Healthcare Providers:

 Regular check-ins with healthcare providers, including endocrinologists, dietitians, and diabetes educators, can help diabetics stay informed about new developments in diabetes management.

 Healthcare providers can also offer personalized advice on how to incorporate fruit into a diabetic diet.

- Online Courses and Webinars:

 Many diabetes organizations and universities offer online courses and webinars on diabetes management, including topics like nutrition, technology, and personalized medicine.

 These resources can be a convenient way to stay informed and continue learning.

- Apps and Online Communities:

 Many apps and online communities for diabetics offer articles, videos, and discussion forums on the latest topics in diabetes management.

 Engaging with these communities can provide valuable insights and support.

The Role of Healthcare Providers in Educating Diabetics About Fruit Consumption

Healthcare providers play a crucial role in educating diabetics about how to manage their diet, including fruit consumption.

By providing personalized guidance and staying up-to-date on the latest research, healthcare providers can help diabetics make informed decisions that support their health.

- Personalized Advice:

 Healthcare providers can offer personalized advice on which fruits to include in a diabetic diet, how to manage portion sizes, and how to pair fruits with other foods to optimize blood sugar control.

 This tailored guidance is essential for helping diabetics navigate the complexities of their diet.

- Ongoing Education:

 Regular appointments with healthcare providers provide an opportunity for ongoing education about diabetes management.

 Providers can share new research, update dietary recommendations, and help diabetics make adjustments to their diet as needed.

- Support and Encouragement:

 In addition to providing information, healthcare providers can offer support and encouragement, helping diabetics stay motivated and confident in their ability to manage their condition.

 This support is especially important when it comes to making dietary changes, which can be challenging.

The Takeaway

 The future of fruit in diabetic diets is bright, with emerging research, advancing technology, and a growing emphasis on personalized nutrition offering new opportunities for diabetics to enjoy fruit while maintaining good blood sugar control.

 By staying informed and taking advantage of the latest tools and resources, diabetics can make empowered choices that support their health and well-being.

As we continue to learn more about diabetes and nutrition, the relationship between fruit and diabetes will likely become even more nuanced, with tailored recommendations that allow for greater flexibility and enjoyment.

Whether through personalized dietary plans, the use of technology, or continued education, diabetics have more tools than ever to navigate the complexities of their diet and live a healthy, balanced life.

Conclusion

The love-hate relationship between fruit and diabetics is complex, but it doesn't have to be a source of stress or anxiety.

By understanding the nutritional benefits and challenges of fruit, making smart choices, and staying informed, diabetics can enjoy the sweetness of fruit without compromising their health.

As we look to the future, the role of fruit in a diabetic diet is likely to become even more central, with new research and technology offering exciting possibilities for personalized nutrition.

With the right knowledge and tools, diabetics can turn the love-hate relationship with fruit into one of balance and harmony, enjoying all the benefits that fruit has to offer as part of a healthy, diabetes-friendly diet.

Please use the next few pages
for your notes and debates.